# How to Lose 10 Pounds in One Week

## They Didn't Think I Could...but I Did!

By Natalie Johnson

# Table of Contents

Introduction

Chapter 1    Setting a Goal                              1

Chapter 2    Your Diet                                   4

Chapter 3    Your Workout                               10

Chapter 4    Simple Ways to Burn Calories               15

Conclusion                                              20

# Introduction

I want to thank you and congratulate you for downloading the book, *"How to Lose 10 Pounds in One Week."*

This book contains proven steps and strategies on how you can successfully shed 10 pounds in such a short period as a week.

Do you have the sudden need to lose ten pounds in just a week? It might be that you are to attend a homecoming dance or you might have been invited to a family reunion. You might even be preparing for the beach season so that you can fit into your sexy swimsuit.

Of course, you would want to look your best on occasions such as these. Well, it is possible to shed ten pounds in just a short amount of time. However, it is not a walk in the park. Losing weight will require a lot of dedication on your part.

Thanks again for downloading this book, I hope you enjoy it!

# Chapter 1
# Setting a Goal

Every journey begins with setting a goal. Right now, your goal is to shed ten pounds in just seven days. In order to lose ten pounds, you need to burn thirty-five thousand calories. Divide that amount by seven days and you end up having to burn at least three thousand calories per day. Now, you have a goal and with that, you already have something to look forward to.

## Should you hire a trainer or not?

Losing ten pounds is definitely a difficult feat. That is why the idea of hiring a trainer might have crossed your mind. It is not that difficult to find a qualified and competent physical trainer. You can easily find one in your local gym or you can check out the newspaper ads. Of course, you can browse the Internet for any available personal trainer in your area. There are a lot of perks in hiring a trainer. Here are some examples.

- Personal trainers can provide a personal program – Wouldn't it be nice if you can engage in a program that is basically designed for your needs? A personal trainer can help you with that. When it comes to weight loss, people have varying needs. For example, there are those who would want to target their abdominal fat while there are those who want sexier legs. Also, a personal trainer can professionally assess you and determine what routines and diet plans would be more suitable for you. This is so that you will be able to lose a whopping 10 pounds in just a week or in the soonest time possible.

- Personal trainers are trained motivators - Another obvious perk in hiring a personal trainer is that he can provide motivation whenever you need it. So many people in the past have tried to lose weight. So many have dreamed of becoming way sexier than they are. But they failed. Why? This is because they lacked motivation, and that is very important. Losing weight on your own can really be boring. Being alone in your journey to weight loss is just like eating by yourself in the cafeteria or even participating in a marathon with no other contestants. Personal trainers are excellent encouragers and they can push you to your limits in order to achieve your goals.

Of course, there are several disadvantages on hiring a trainer as well. For example, there is the cost. Personal trainers do not offer their services for free. You would really have to invest in order to benefit from them. Another probable disadvantage is that you might not develop a good relationship with your trainer. Having a good relationship between the trainer and trainee is important. After all, he would be the one who would accompany you in your journey to weight loss.

The decision to hire a trainer is yours to make. Whether or not you choose to work with a professional in your weight loss training would have to depend on what you feel comfortable with and what would ultimately motivate you to push harder towards your weight loss goal.

# Chapter 2
# Your Diet

Losing ten pounds in a week requires you to focus on two major aspects – diet and exercise. Both are very crucial especially if you want to lose a huge amount of weight in a very short time. Now, if you browse online, you will find a lot of dietary plans out there. Some are proven to be effective while some are very dangerous.

One of those things that you should definitely not try is crash dieting. Crash dieting refers to that old weight loss method where one severely prevents himself from taking calories. Most crash dieters reach even the point of starvation just so they would not 'add more fats' to their body. Crash dieting seems to be a logical way for anyone who does not want to get fat. But it is very dangerous.

First of all, crash dieters deprive themselves from the nutritional benefits that they can get from foods. Second, most crash dieters find themselves in a vicious cycle of weight gain and weight loss. Once they successfully lose a huge amount of weight, they end up reverting back to their old eating habits. Usually, the weight they were able to gain during that period is more than the weight they lost while on their crash diet.

Crash dieting can cause malnutrition, can make you look older than your age, and can definitely put your health at risk. Thus, you should never try it. Read on to have a better grasp of how to control your food intake.

## Counting calories

So how can you lose a lot of weight if you are not allowed to starve yourself? Well, this is where counting calories comes in. These days, almost all food products come with a nutritional fact sheet. The fact sheet will let you determine not only how much calories you can gain from that product but what kinds of vitamins you can get from it as well. Contrary to popular belief, calories are important in helping you lose weight. Because it is from calories where you get energy for your physical exercises. Without calories, you would get very weak and perform poorly when doing weight loss routines.

Later on, you will learn how to effectively burn the calories that you take. But first, you might want to familiarize yourself with the following low-calorie foods that you might want to include in your diet.

- Celery – If there is one food that you will grow to love as you try to lose weight, it will definitely be celery. It only contains five calories per stem. Thus, you can eat lots of it without having to worry about gaining weight.

Now, there are a lot of ways to enjoy celery. You can always eat it after washing it. But traditionally, people dip their celery in cheese and even in mayonnaise. But such dairy products contain a lot of fat. If you want a flavorful celery treat, you can always dip it in Dijon mustard or even chili sauce for a healthier snack.

- Broccoli – Broccoli is probably one of the most despised vegetables out there. Even if you are one of those who do not like it, you might start loving it once you find out about how it can help you lose weight. A cup of broccoli only contains twenty-five calories. But the good news does not end there. It takes about fifty-five calories to digest that amount of broccoli. So just by consuming broccoli, you can burn fifty-five calories or even more!

- Pepper – Another low-calorie vegetable that you should add to your weight loss diet is pepper. Pepper can always be an additional ingredient to spice up your meals for your seven days of dieting. Eating pepper would cause your body to produce heat as well as increase oxygen consumption for twenty minutes. These cause your body to burn more calories. It would be a lot better for you to eat ripe pepper. This is because the riper a pepper becomes, the more nutrition it offers. If you want, you can always eat pepper raw.

- Spinach – If you grew up in the eighties or even in the nineties, you might have watched Popeye eat his spinach and become supernaturally strong. Though spinach does not actually give you super strength, it can help you lose weight fast. You can always enjoy a spinach salad topped with tomatoes and chopped onions. If you want, you have a spinach smoothie as well – a more refreshing snack than ice cream. Like other leafy greens, spinach is also very rich in fiber.

- Cranberries – Of course, for your diet week, you might crave for sweets. Well, instead of reaching for a sugar-laden chocolate bar, you might want to go for cranberries instead. They are very flavorful, but you do not have to worry about that because they are very low in sugar. Also, cranberries are high in fiber. Foods that are high in fiber are important in losing weight because they help improve digestion and prevent constipation. Aside from contributing to weight loss, cranberries also have amazing anti-cancer properties.

- Grapefruit – Studies have shown that people who have eaten grapefruit while trying to lose weight were able to lose weight more than those who did not eat grapefruit. Thus, there is no harm in adding this fruit in your diet especially if you have grown tired of cranberries. This fruit can definitely supply the nutrients that a dieter really needs. It contains potassium, vitamin C, beta-carotene, and antioxidants. With grapefruit, you can get the nutrients you need for the day without having to consume a lot of calories.

- Apricots – Next, there are apricots. For every one hundred gram of apricots you only get fifty calories. The good thing about apricots is that they can really help you feel full. That is why there are a perfect breakfast treat. Two pieces of medium-sized apricots usually contains about a gram and a half of fiber. Apricots are also rich in numerous vitamins and nutrients and these include potassium, vitamin A, and others that help fight cancers as well as heart disease.

- Chicken – If you are like the numerous others who cannot live the life of a vegetarian, you would definitely crave for meat. But be careful about the type of meat you eat especially since red meat is high in calories as well as cholesterol. Thus, you might want to go for chicken. Boiling or steaming chicken are the best preparation methods for dieters who want to lose weight. Frying your chicken might make it very delicious. But fried chicken can be very oily and that is not good for any person trying to lose weight.

- Oatmeal – Of course, a weight loss aspirant's diet can never be complete without oatmeal. Oatmeal can help prevent constipation and does not contain anything that will make you fat. It is packed with energy so you can eat it if you are to do some exhaustive workouts later in the day. Also, oatmeal can easily make you feel full. Thus, the tendencies to overeat are reduced.

It is important for you to burn at least 3,500 calories a day. But of course, you have to add your daily food intake to this amount too. If you are to consume, say, one thousand calories for a certain day, then you would have to at burn at least 4,500 calories. The amount of calories you burn should be 3,500 calories more than the amount you plan to take for the day. Thus, weight loss can be achieved easier if you choose to eat foods with fewer calories.

There are numerous software as well as websites that can help you count your calories. Some of these are free, while you might also be interested in the ones available for certain rates. You might consider investing in these since they can help you track your calories burned at a more precise rate.

# Chapter 3
# Your Workout

Now comes the other important aspect of weight loss which is exercise. You must have a very good workout plan so that you will be able to burn all those fats that make you very heavy. Anyone who wants to lose ten pounds in a week must engage in both cardiovascular and strength training. Here are some examples of activities that you have to do for a week to lose ten pounds.

**Top calorie-burning activities**

- Jumping rope – The most exhaustive and most effective calorie-burning activity that you can engage in is jumping rope. Jumping rope is not just an activity for those little girls playing by the side walk. In fact, professional athletes such as boxers and runners include jumping rope in their daily routines. In just thirty minutes of jumping rope, you can actually burn more than four hundred calories. Now, jumping rope can be quite tricky. But practice makes perfect.

- Running – The next top activity that can help you lose weight fast is running. Running for thirty minutes at a steady pace can help you lose more than four hundred calories. Of course, if you have been running before, then you might want to run for about an hour or so. Some people can burn at least one thousand and five hundred calories in an hour. Most people prefer jogging early in the morning when the weather is cool and there are not enough cars on the street. For the seven days wherein you will try to lose weight, you must set four running schedules for at least four days.

- Rowing – Rowing has always been considered as an awesome sport perfect for weight loss aspirants. Rowing will mostly involve your abdominal muscles as well as your upper body muscles. So if you want flat abs, a firm chest, and a pair of guns for arms, then this is a sport that you can always try out. Rowing vigorously for thirty minutes can help you lose three hundred calories.

- Stair-climbing – At this point, you might want to start hating escalators and elevators. This is because stair-climbing can help you lose weight fast as well. Climbing up the stairs will help strengthen your lower muscles and make it free from fat. If you go to the stadium, you might see some individuals climbing up and down the stadium steps. You might want to join them. If climbing up and down the stairs gets boring, you can always spice up your routine by taking two steps at a time or even jumping a step using two feet at a time.

- Swimming – Another awesome activity to consider is swimming. Freestyle swims can help you burn up to three hundred calories in half an hour. The good thing about swimming is that it involves almost every major muscle group. Thus, it can provide an overall workout for your body. Swimming is perfect especially if you want your muscles toned by the end of the week. A word of caution – never swim alone.

There are still numerous activities out there that can help you lose weight fast. For example, you can always get busy with sports such as soccer, basketball, or even volleyball. It is very important to allot a certain period every day for a physical activity.

## Keep dehydrated

It is very important to keep hydrated. The physical routines mentioned earlier can really be exhausting. Your body will definitely lose a lot of water. Thus, you have to make sure that your body fluids are replenished. Stick to water as much as possible rather than juices, coffee, and other sugary drinks. If you want, you can opt for those sugar-free energy drinks in case you need an extra boost for your workout sessions. But do not drink too much of these as they have side effects – they might cause you to go sleepless or they might cause you to be cranky for the whole day.

## Do not tire yourself out

It is normal to get tired after every workout session. Do not commit that mistake of spending all of your time working out. Your body is not a machine that can continue working for seven days. It needs to rest too. You have to rest so that your muscles can recover and be ready for you next strenuous workout. It is very dangerous for your health to keep going even when your body could not continue any longer.

When you tire yourself too much, there is always that chance for you to have very low sugar levels causing you to lose your consciousness at any given moment. There have been cases of individuals passing out while they are jogging or even by simply sitting and watching TV after a hard day's workout. Working out too much can also cause dehydration.

## Never fail to do warm-ups and cool-downs

Warm-ups and cool-downs are very important. If you own a car, you do not step on the gas pedal right away, do you? And if you are a singer, you do not directly hitting those very high notes, do you? Warm-ups are very important not only in starting a car or singing but also in doing physical work-outs. You have to stretch your muscles first. Stretching your muscles can help reduce cramps later on. After you do some stretches, you have to do some light movements such as jogging in place, doing some jumping jacks, or even doing some air jobs. You have to make your muscles all warmed-up and ready for intense calorie-burning routines.

And do not forget to do some cool-downs as well. You do not just drop down on the ground or even sit down after doing some push-ups for instance. Automatically resting after an intense routine can cause complications in your blood flow and even raise the risks of a heart attack. Cool-down routines are basically the same as warm-up routines – light jogs, jumping jacks, and air jabs.

# Chapter 4
# Simple Ways to Burn Calories

As mentioned earlier, you do not always have to be in your workout attire and breaking sweat just to lose weight. There are a number of simple ways on how you can burn calories easily. Here are some examples:

- Watch a funny TV show – How can watching a funny TV show help you burn calories? Well, they say that laughter is the best medicine. It turns out that laughter can also help you lose weight. Whenever you laugh, the abdominal muscles contract. Thus, whenever you watch a funny TV show, you can basically give your abdomen a nice workout. Just make sure you do not sit in front of the TV for hours.

- Have a hot shower then soak in cold water– Did you know that hot showers can help you lose weight faster? Studies show that hot water can help contribute to weight loss. Having a hot shower can help increase your metabolic rate. Hot water helps you work out a sweat. Now, you might want to try what other people do after a hot shower and that is soaking in cold water. Experts are still debating regarding the effect of hot and cold water in bathing. However, there is no harm in trying.

- Sit and meditate – Whenever you get stressed, your tendency to gain weight gets higher. Thus, you should never let yourself get stressed out. If you find your mind clogged up with so many things, you can always sit down in a corner and meditate. To help you meditate better, you can always play soothing music from the Internet. Sound effects like chirping crickets and babbling brooks can also help you get into a meditative stated.

- Drink tea – Have you ever wondered why most people of Southeast Asia, especially in the northern province of China, are not obese? Well, this is because most Southeast Asians love to drink tea after a very hearty meal. Teas are consumed even during lazy afternoons. Tea is a laxative and it can also help boost your metabolism. Opt for green tea instead of black tea.

**Example of a weight loss week**

Using everything that you have learned, your diet week schedule might end up being something like this schedule of Bob – a fictitious person also trying to lose weight:

- Sunday – Bob wakes up early in the morning and decides to engage in a physical activity. He has not worked out before so a strenuous workout routine is not advisable at the moment. He decides to do something that he will enjoy in a nice Sunday morning and that is swimming at the lake. After swimming, Bob felt very hungry. It is a good thing that there was still some left over spinach at the refrigerator. For lunch and supper, Bob feasted on fruits and vegetables like apricots and grapefruit.

- Monday- Monday morning begins and Bob has to go to work early. For his breakfast. Bob ate a healthy green salad consisting of broccoli, celery, and spinach. At work, Bob sees the elevator broken so he decides to take the stairs letting him burn calories in the process. By the end of the day, Bob successfully finished work and he headed straight to the gym so that he can run on the treadmill.

- Tuesday- For this day, Bob has decided to wake up an hour earlier than usual so that he can jog in the morning. He was able to jog around his neighborhood for thirty minutes and he was able to burn five hundred calories already. For breakfast, Bob had oatmeal partnered with low-fat milk. At the end of the day, Bob went home early to engage in high intensity training using a workout video he downloaded online as a guide. After training and eating a low-calorie meal, Bob was invited by his friends to play basketball right away. Thus, Bob was able to burn more weight before the night ended.

- Wednesday – For the fourth day of dieting, Bob suddenly grew tired of eating fruits. His body is now craving for meat. After thirty minutes of jogging, he cooked some chicken breasts stored in the freezer, ate it and finished off his breakfast with a spinach smoothie. The afternoon got a little lazy. It was a good thing that Bob's workplace has a tennis court and he played with his co-workers for an hour. After work, Bob hurriedly went home, put on his running shoes and did a few rounds around the neighborhood.

- Thursday – On Thursday, things got a little bit busy at work and Bob found himself very stressed out. He felt the urge to pig out. But since he was on a diet, he had fruits for lunch instead. He was able to feel relieved as nutrients from the fruits were able to reenergize him. From Monday until now, Bob has always taken the stairs making his leg muscles a lot stronger than before. Because he was too stressed, Bob was not able to run for that day. But he was relieved from stress after sipping a few cups of tea.

- Friday – Thank God it's Friday! Getting enough sleep from last night, Bob woke up early in the mornings so that he can run again. He was able to pass by a group of kids playing soccer and they asked him to join them. Not only did Bob enjoy playing soccer but he was also able to burn a lot. For this final day of work for the week, Bob ate celery dipped in delicious Dijon mustard. On his way home later on, he was approached by Sally, a pretty co-worker and she invited her to a Zumba session for the next day. Bob agreed.

- Saturday – Saturday morning came and Bob woke up very excited. He feels a lot better, a lot slimmer, and a lot better-looking. This is due to the fact that he has eaten nothing but healthy foods for the week and he was able to do a lot of physical activities to keep him strong and healthy. After Zumba classes, Bob took Sally to a Vegetarian restaurant where they were able to eat low-calorie meals. Sally complimented Bob on how good-looking he is. Inspired, Bob did some push-ups and aerobic routines once he arrived at home.

Throughout the week Bob was able to burn three thousand calories every day. You will see that it is not really impossible to lose weight fast.

# Conclusion

Thank you again for downloading this book!

I hope this book was able to help you to get a clearer idea of how you can lose ten pounds in just a week. As mentioned earlier, you would have to exert a lot of dedication if you want to achieve your weight loss goal.

Always seek to burn three thousand pounds or more in a day and you will definitely be ready for a day at a beach or a night at your homecoming party or family reunion. The next step is to get started on your 1-week plan.

Finally, if you enjoyed this book, please take the time to share your thoughts and post a review on Amazon. It'd be greatly appreciated!

Thank you and good luck!